SWAMI CAT SAYS
Words of Wisdom to Purr By

Edited by Yoga Girl
Illustrations by Nitya Martino

Text Copyright © 2013 by Lynne Elson
Illustrations copyright © 2013 by Nitya Martino

Published by:
Elson Enterprises
LynneElson.com

Preface:

For a little bit of time during my stray kitten phase, I didn't listen to my teachers. I wanted freedom, but didn't know how to get it. I ran away, lived in a cardboard box, ate tuna directly out of the can, (Momma used to say not to because I'd cut my tongue and she was right) I played with the party animals at night and learned how to fend for myself only.

Soon I was sleeping with one eye open, losing all my fur and wasn't enjoying life. When I found my Guru, Sri Purranandaji, I couldn't help but purr. I realized the one thing that was missing was a sense of purr-pose.

My purr-pose is to teach Yoga to anybody, whether human, dog, fish, ferret, aardvark or any other species of animal.

We are all in need of a little scratch behind the ears to remind us that we are loved and can love, unconditionally. We can make this love a peace umbrella to weather the storms that life throws down upon us. And isn't it better to share this umbrella than to keep it all to ourselves? So much more fun. Isn't it so? This is Yoga.

An excerpt from Swami Cat's speech at the opening of the Yoga Magazine Conference Tabby Town, Colorado September 24, 2007

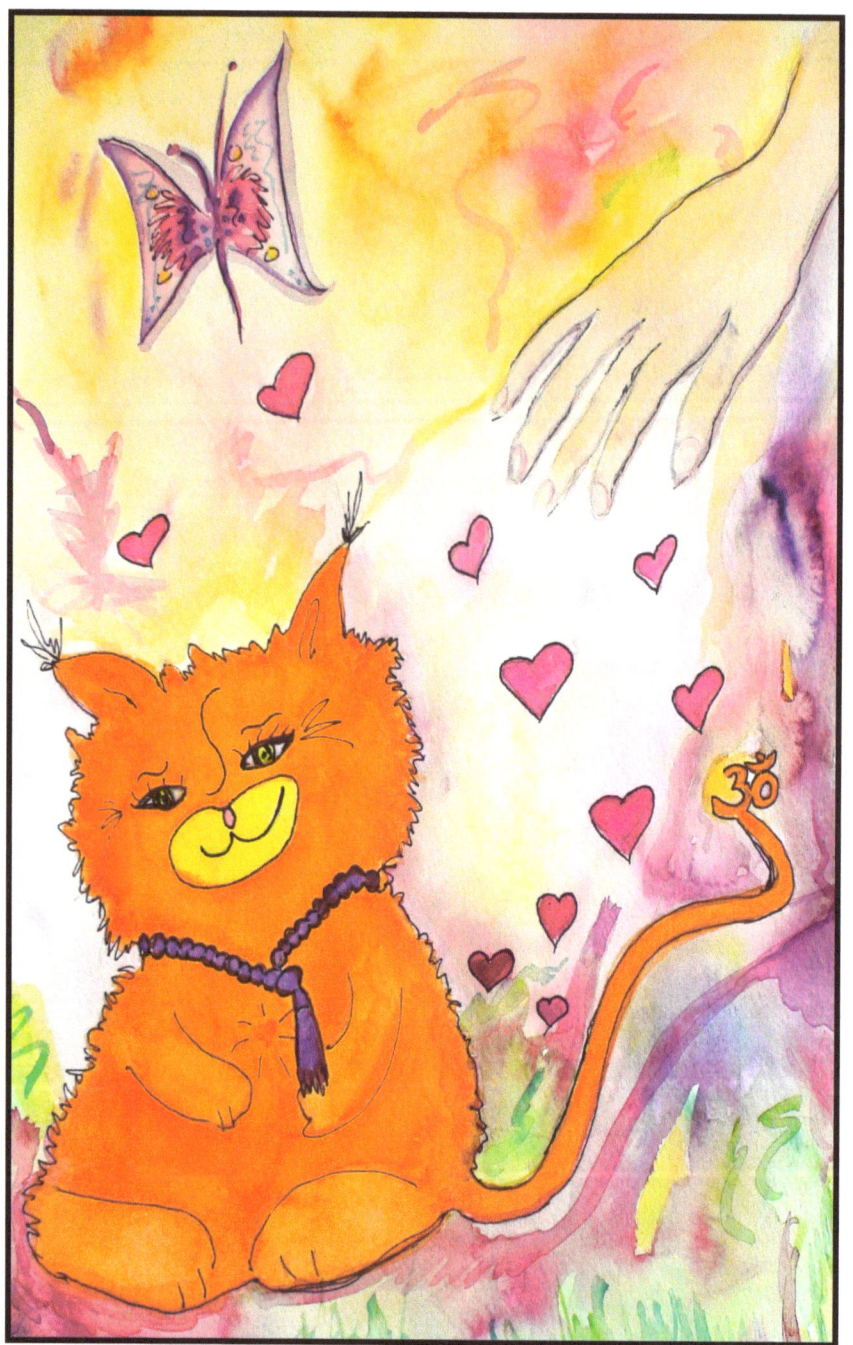

Swami Cat's mantra, "Live for the sake of others."

"Best way to happiness? Count your blessings."

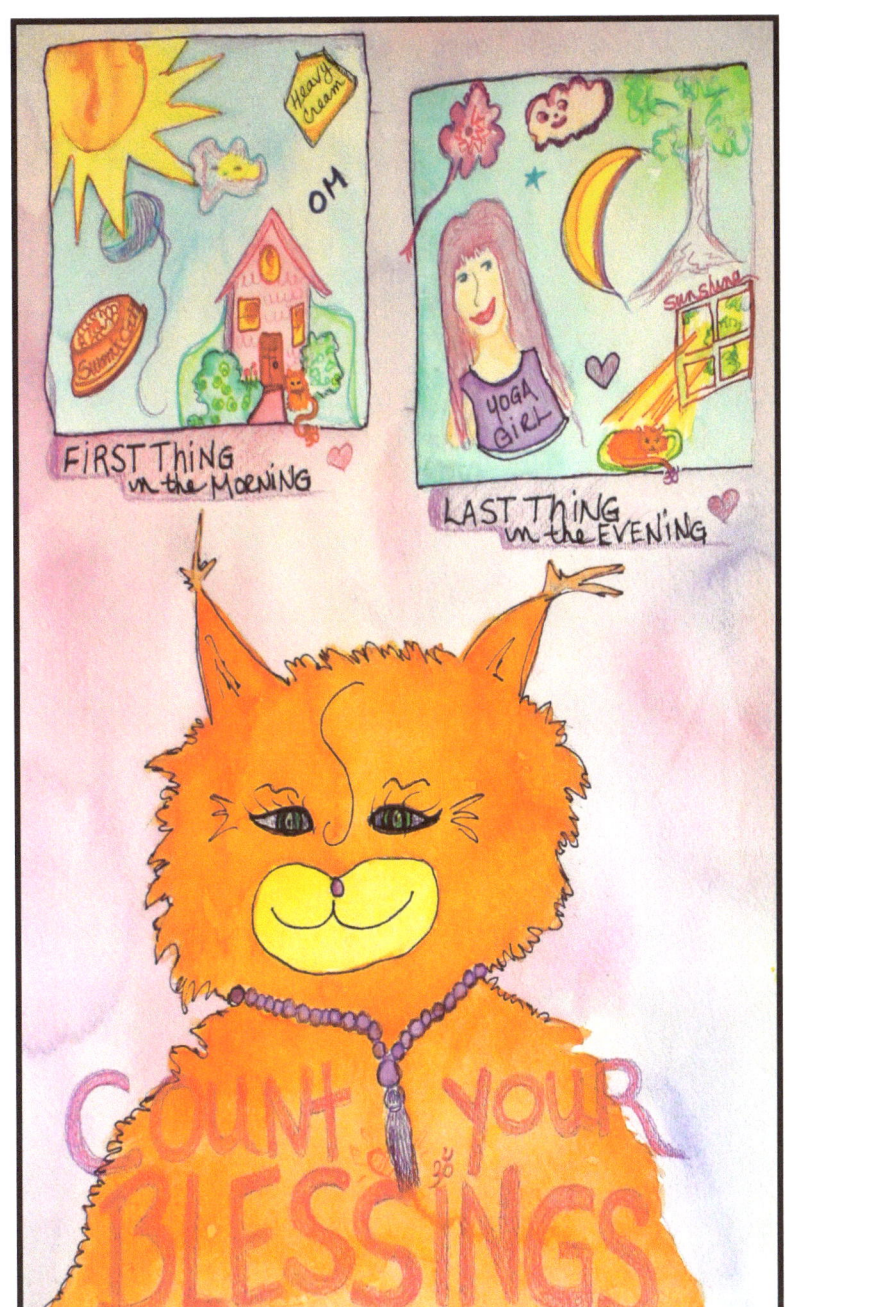

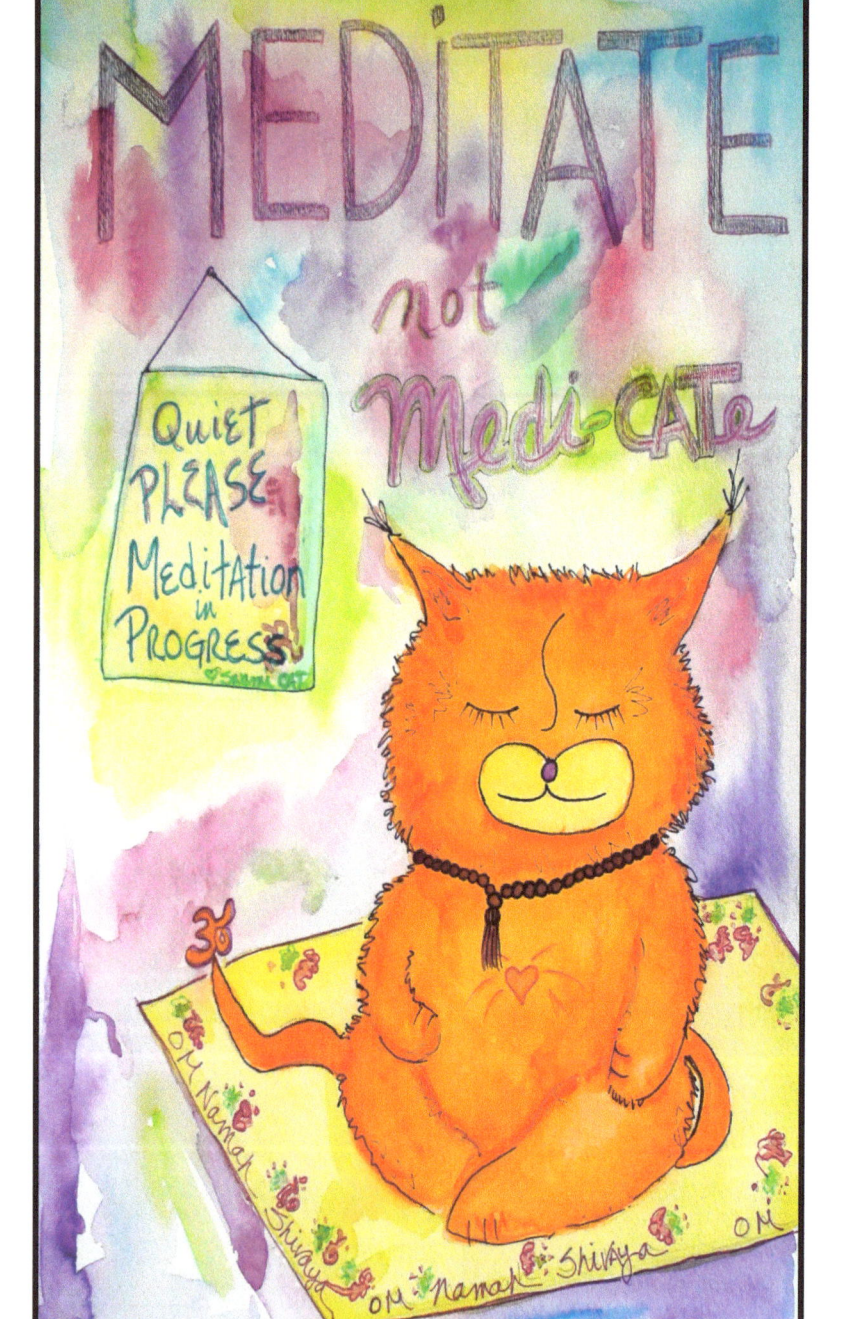

"Try meditation before medication."

"I used to be afraid to go to sleep, but now I take a deep breath and do my Yoga relaxation. Then I can dream that a cat can be president or fly to the moon!"

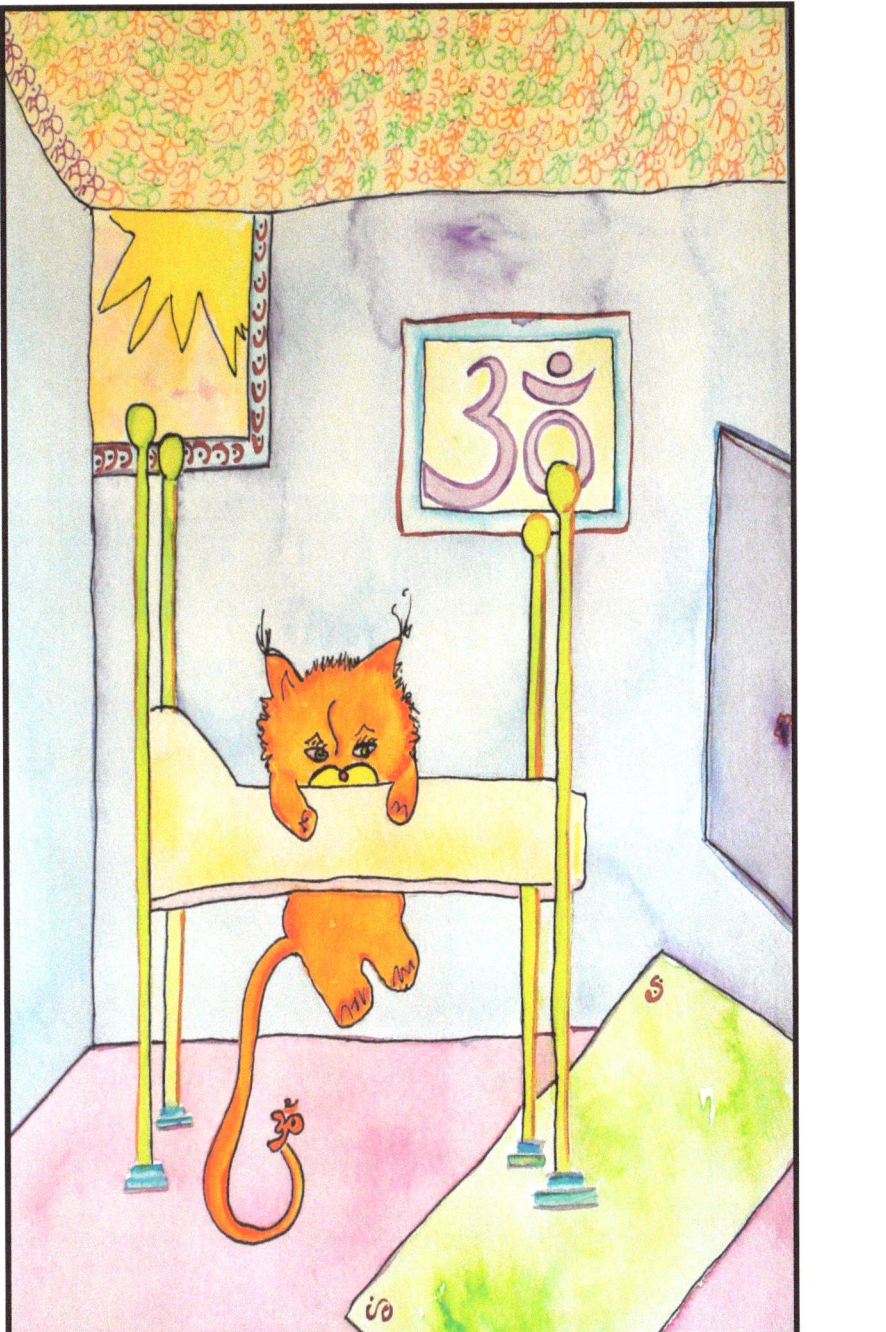

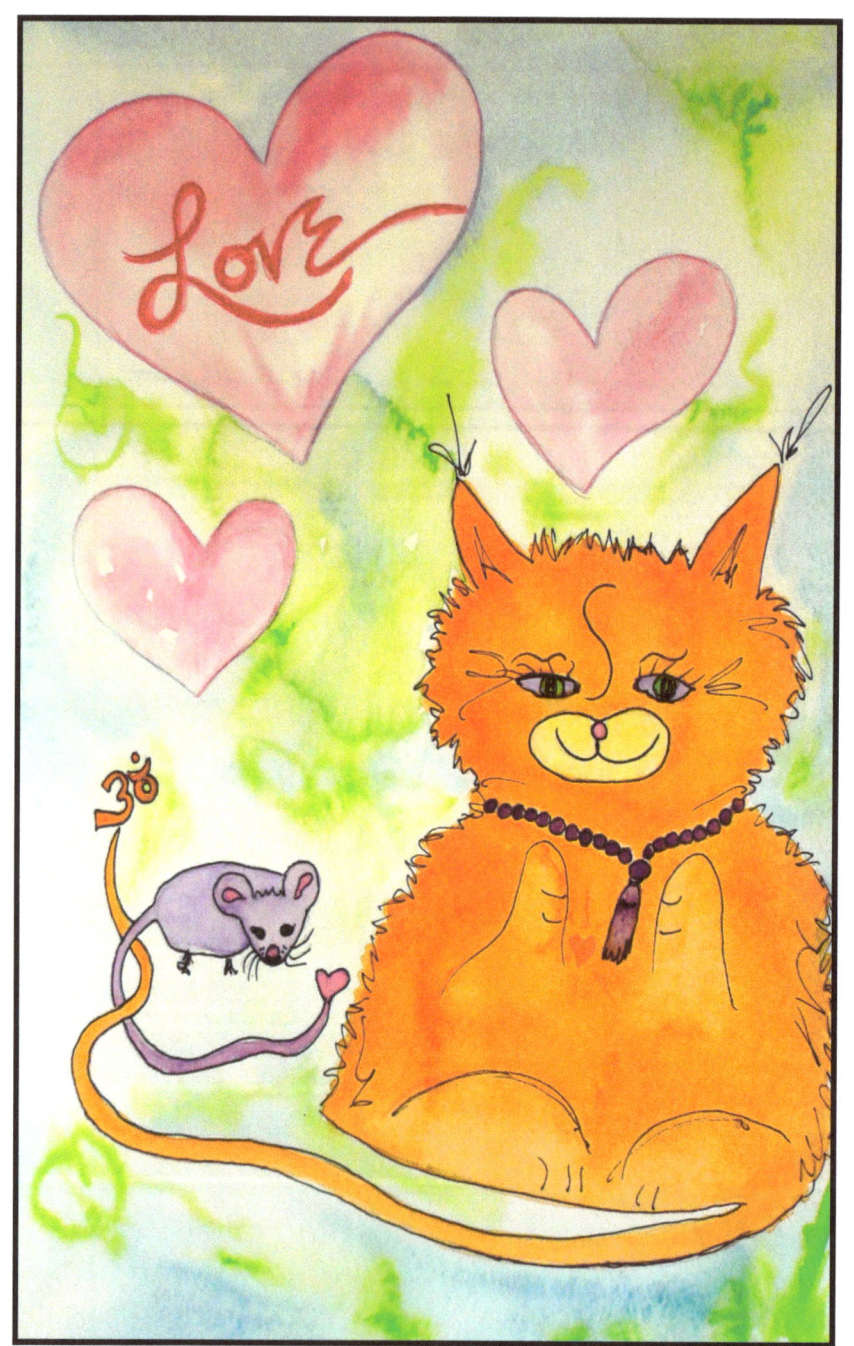

"Love: the antidote to fear."

"Snuggle up to the sunny spot."

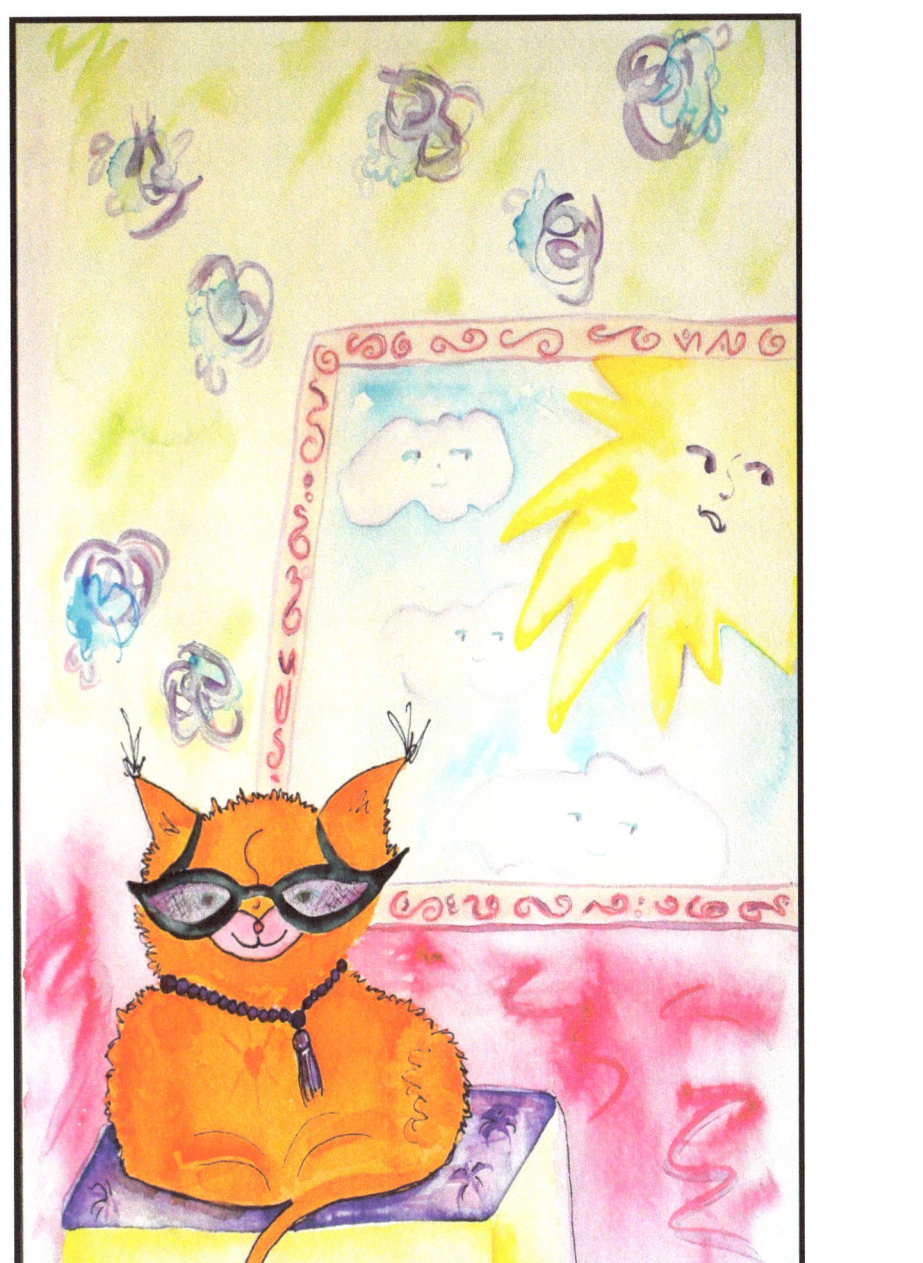

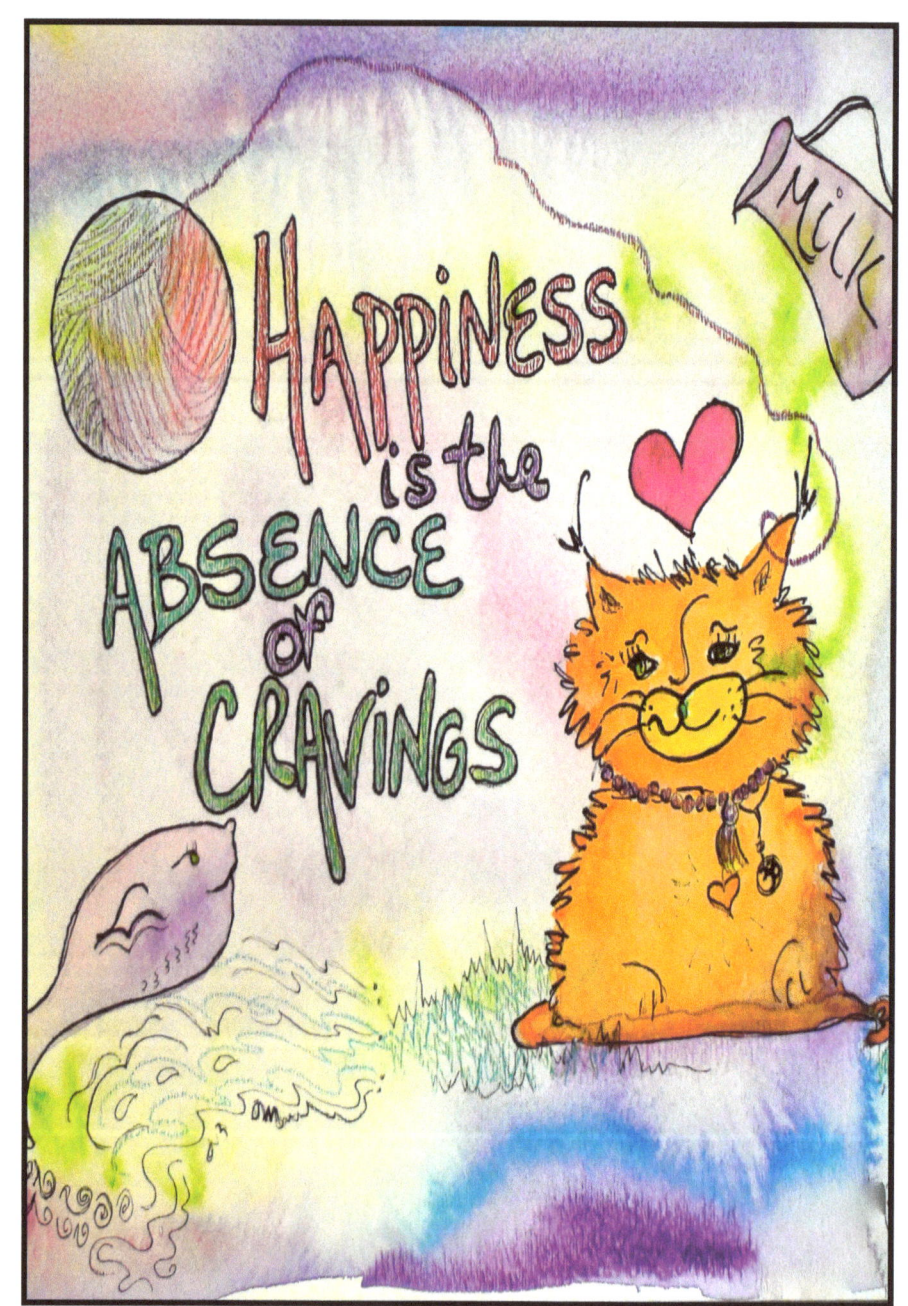

"Before Yoga, I couldn't resist warm milk and a ball of yarn. But now I know, you don't need *things* to make you happy. *Things* only make you happy for a few minutes. Long lasting happiness comes from inside you."

"Yoga is a science. When you practice, you get results."

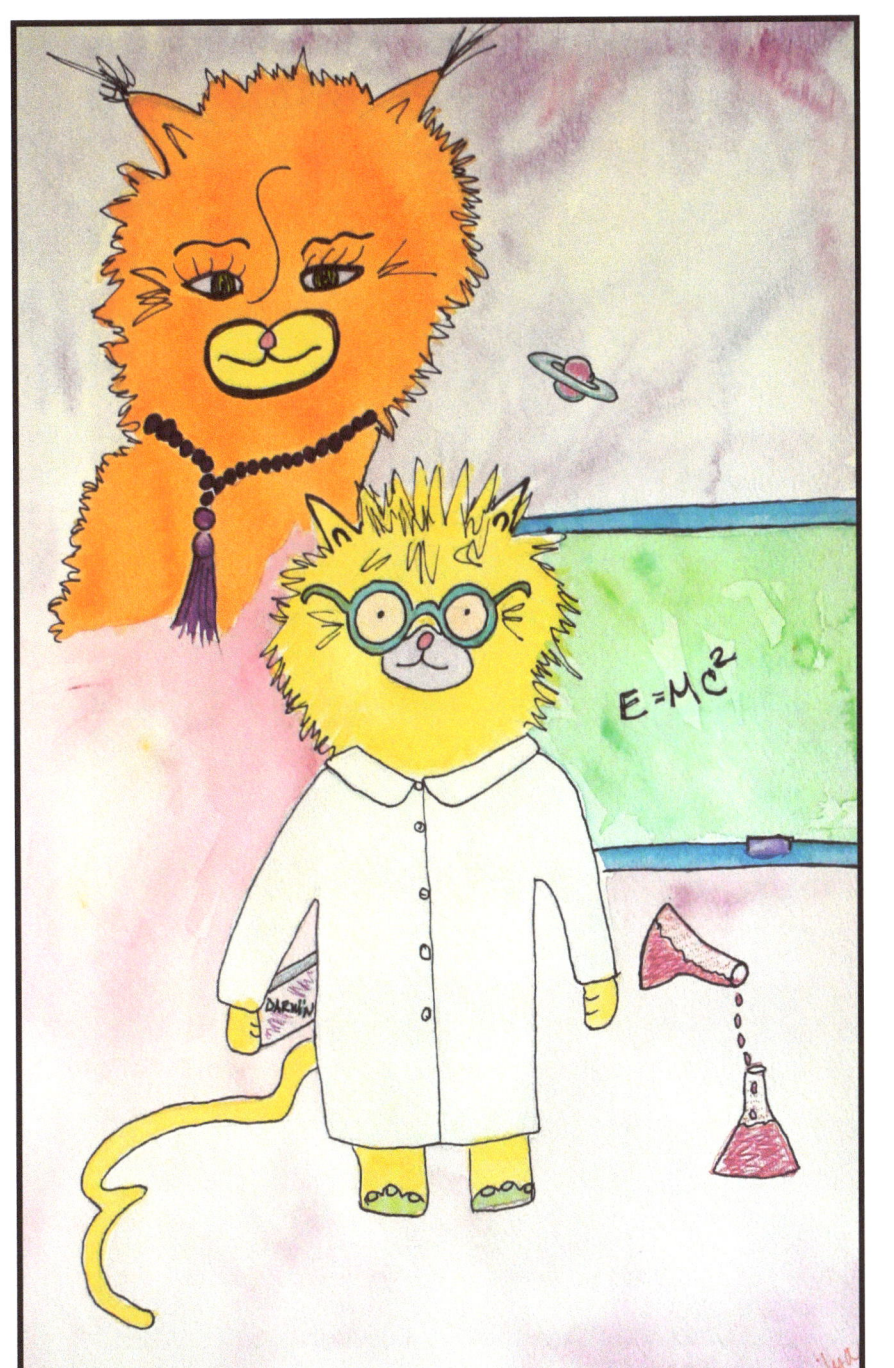

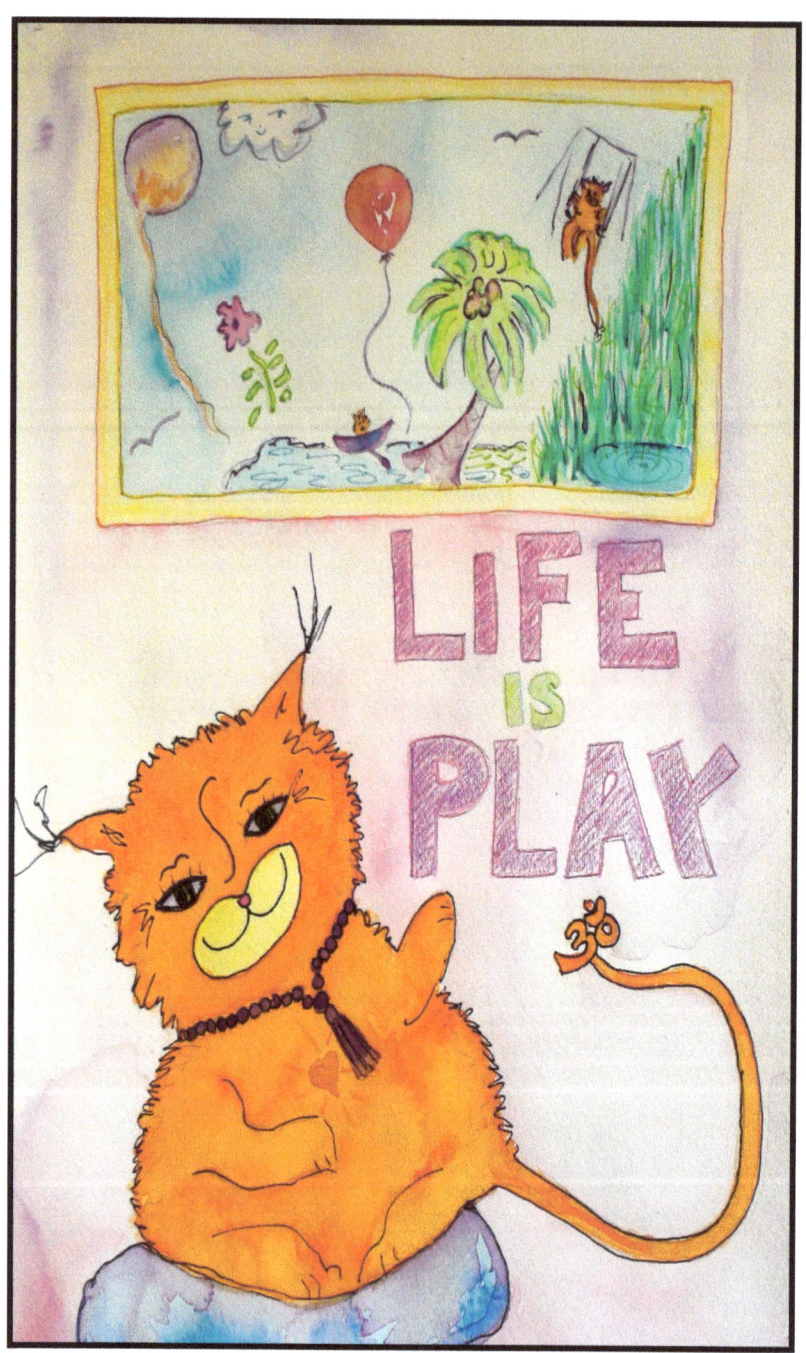

Yoga reminds Swami Cat to enjoy life. "Playing is cat-ageous!"

"Let negativity roll off you, like rain off a slicker."

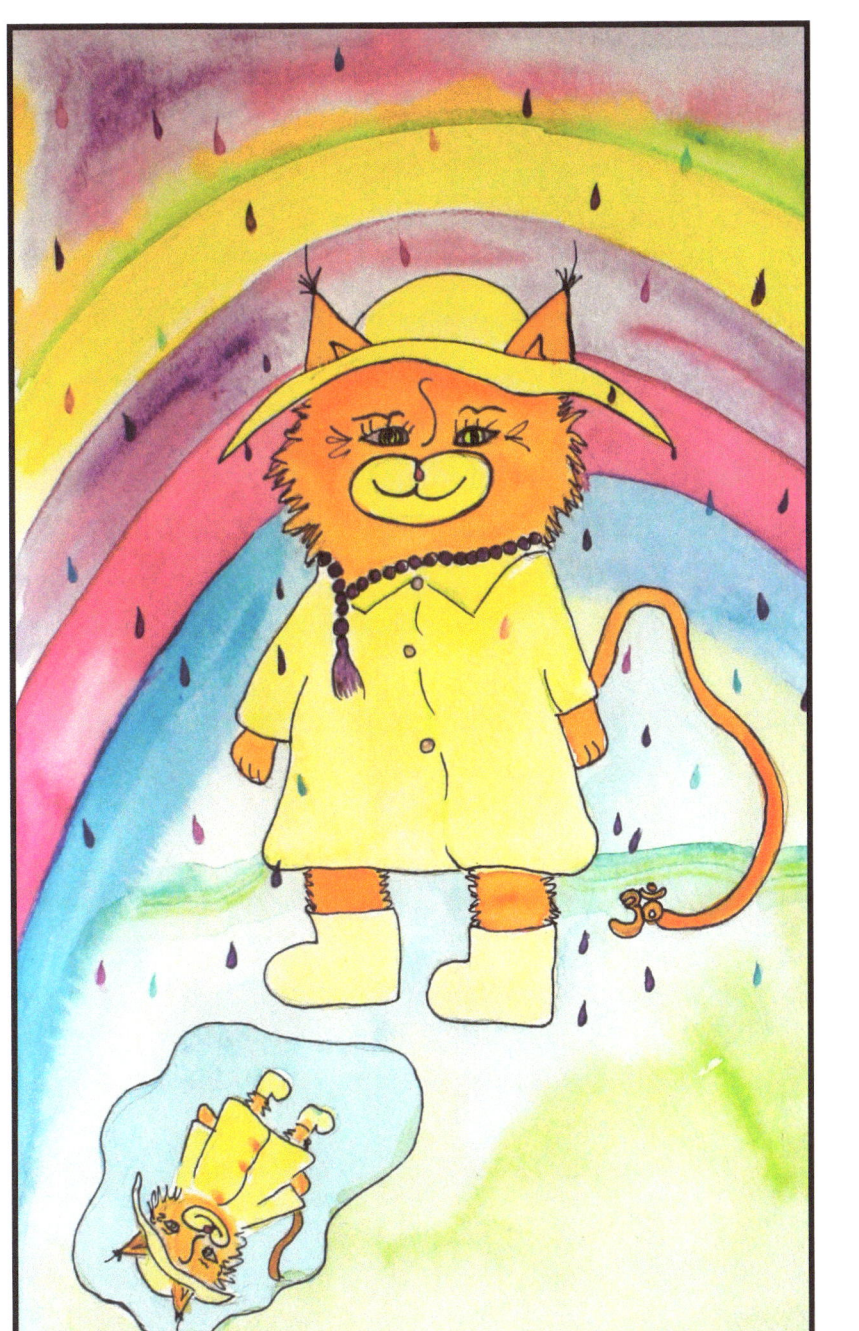

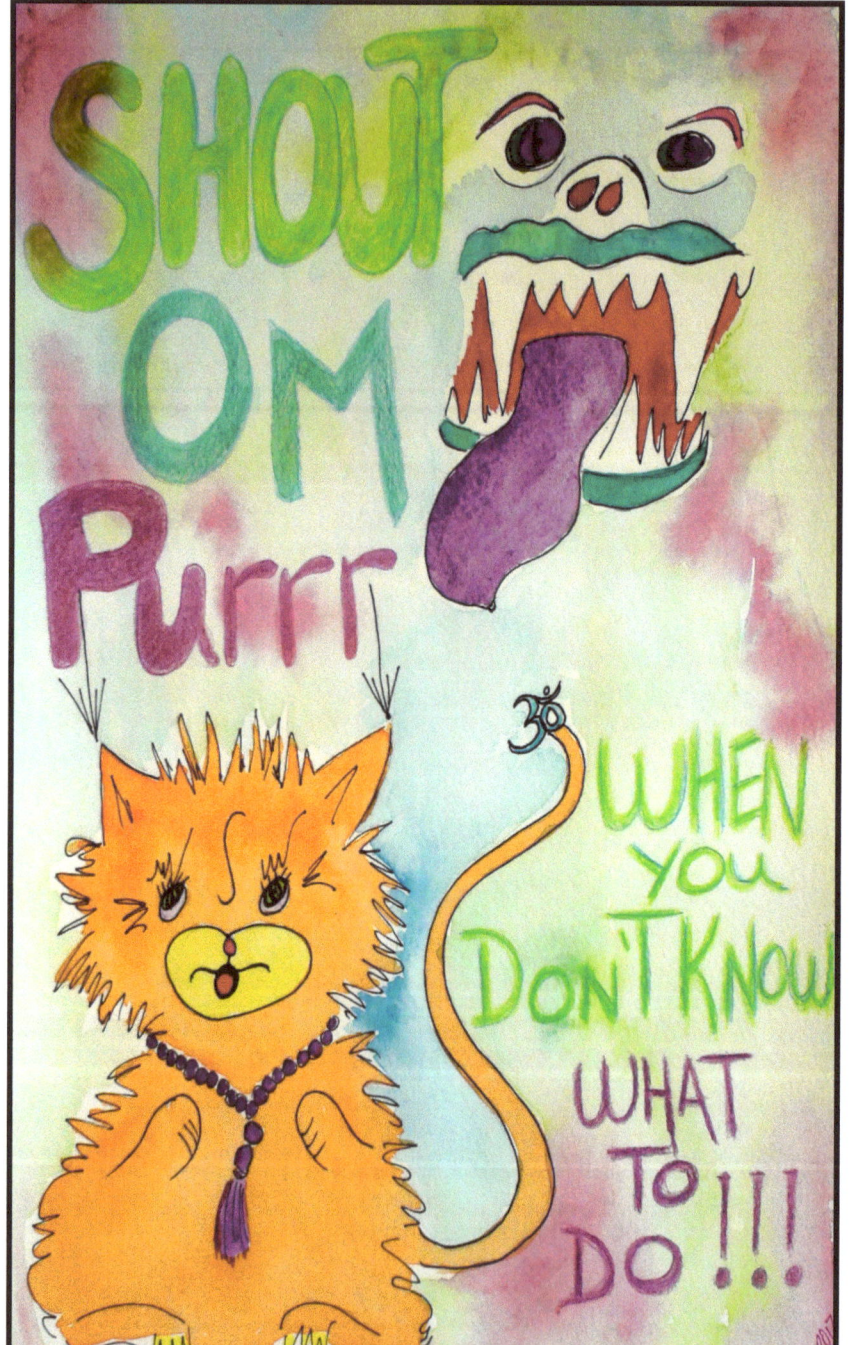

"I shout Om Purr!" at the top of my lungs. That usually scares away all my scary thoughts."

"You are never alone when you practice Yoga. Hundreds of thousands of humans, cats, dogs and fish are stretching, breathing and Om-ing with you."

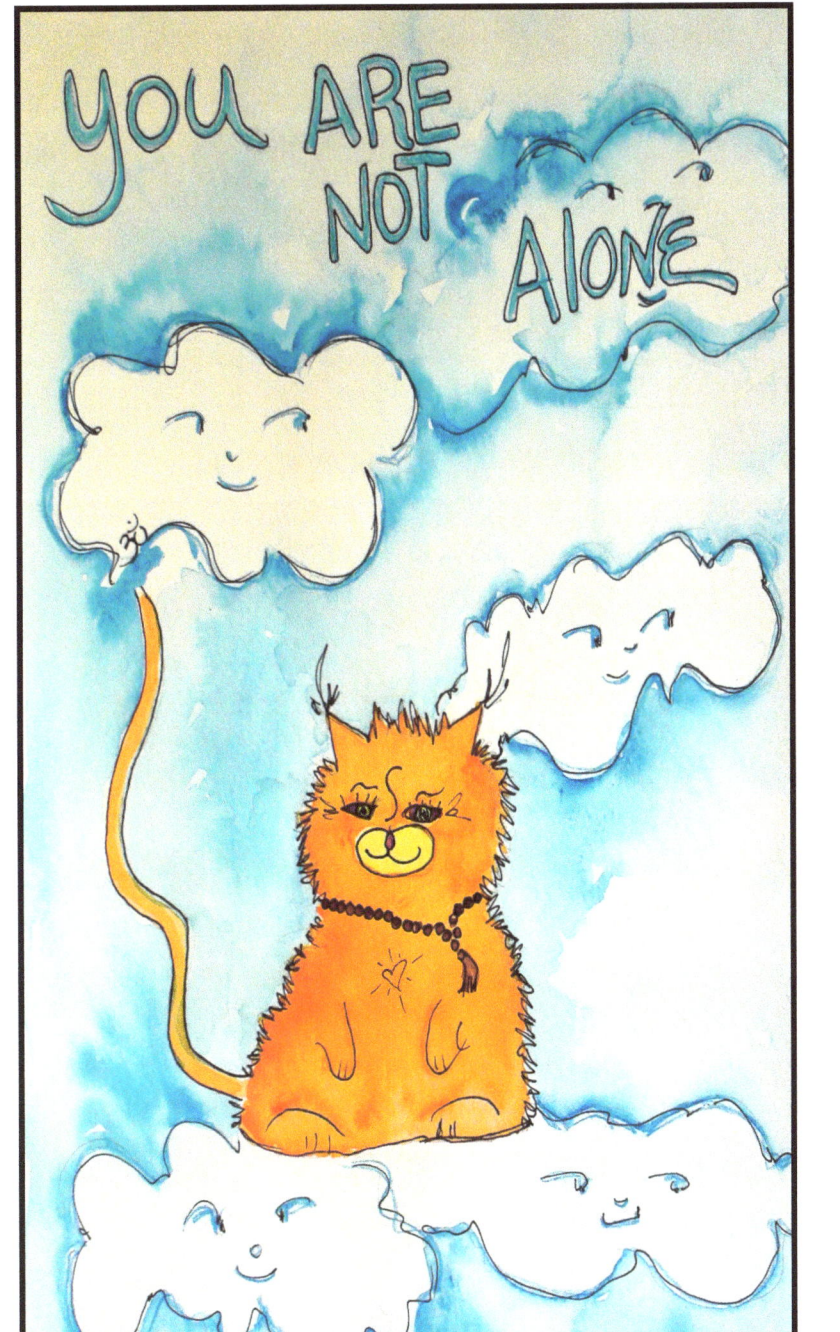

Swami Cat's Quick Yoga Fix

Sometimes someone or something makes you upset. Practicing Yoga every day helps you stay happy inside, no matter what happens to you on the outside. If you still need a quick Yoga fix try one or all of the following:

1. Do some deep Yogic breaths.

2. Sing songs like *Cat's In The Cradle, What's New Pussy Cat* or chant a Yoga song.

3. Pray for all creatures on the planet that are in need of healing and hugs today.

4. Take a meditation walk outside to appreciate all of nature's beautiful miracles: A ladybug crawling on a leaf, a bird eating a berry, a flower opening up its petals.

5. Practice a few sun salutations.

6. Laugh. Watch a funny video or read a funny book. Even if you don't want to laugh at first, just do it. You can trick your brain into feeling better. Try it. It really does work.

7. Pick up garbage as you walk. It makes you and the planet feel better.

Bios:

Swami Cat was born to a large litter in Purramus, New Jersey and named Bob. In his teenage years a lovely young feline performer who had just received a small role in the touring company of a famous Broadway show distracted him. She was kicked out when they realized she was a real cat, but the showbiz bug had already bitten Bob. He dropped out of Garfield High and took off as a roadie, learning many skills including how to take a catnap anywhere. For a while Bob was the lead singer and bass player of a band he formed called Heavy Cream. Bob took up hiking and ended up becoming the first domesticated cat to climb Annapurrna, the 10th largest mountain in the world. Up on the mountaintop he saw a flash of the furry face that would change his life: Swami Purrananda. He then took off for the remote village of Litterahari, which loosely translates as litter box to the Gods. Bob ran into the temple in the middle of the holy ritual of I AMs (of which one of Swami Purrananda's disciples created a very lucrative cat food.) Sri Swami Purranandaji saw him and said, "Ah there you are. I've been waiting for you." Swami Cat was a quick study of the Vedas and soon became head of the "KT's" (kitten trainees). Sri Swami Cat now teaches Yoga to all species of animals, including humans and creates short videos with Yoga Girl about having fun in life through Yoga and meditation.

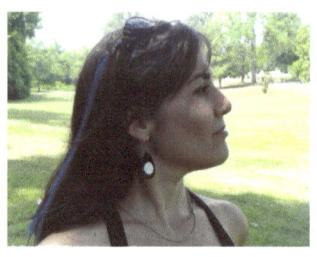

Yoga Girl (A.K.A. Karuna Lynne) is a playwright and teacher of theatre and Yoga. She is a long-time member of the Yoga Life Society. She is eternally grateful for Grandma Irene, who taught her the joy of laughter and creativity, and to Guruji Rev. Jaganath Carrera who inspired her to join her two loves: Yoga and writing. LynneElson.com

Nitya Martino is a certified Structural Yoga Therapist, Yoga teacher, stress management instructor and reflexologist and always an artist for humanity. artandsoul108.com

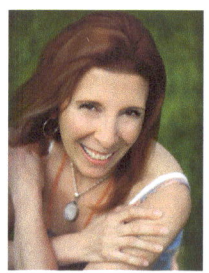

A portion of the proceeds of this book will be lovingly donated to The Yoga Life Society.

www.yogalifesociety.com

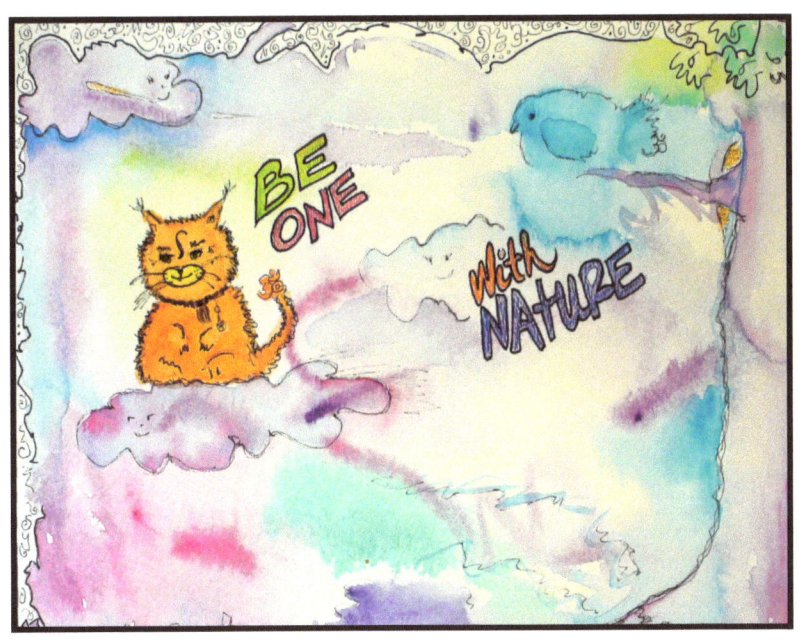

Want more of Swami Cat's playful Yogic sayings,
songs and videos?

Log onto Swamicat.com.

www.ingramcontent.com/pod-product-compliance
Lightning Source LLC
Chambersburg PA
CBHW050921290526
45792CB00002B/836